HUDDLE UP!

A COACH'S PLAYBOOK TO PROGRAM SUCCESS

THOMASINA 'COACH G' GATSON

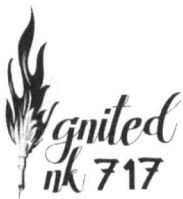

Ignited Ink 717

I

II

CONTENTS

PRE-GAME   3

CHAPTER I: JUMP BALL   7

CHAPTER II: PHILOSOPHY OF COACHING ATHLETICS   15

CHAPTER III: BEYOND THE COURT   22

CHAPTER IV: ETHICS AND SPORTSMANSHIP   37

CHAPTER V: LEGAL ASPECTS AND CONSIDERATIONS   44

CHAPTER VI: PROGRAM DEVELOPMENT   53

CHAPTER VII: PSYCHOLOGY OF COACHING   88

CHAPTER VIII: ATS FOR COACHING BASKETBALL   94

CHAPTER IX: AT THE BUZZER   105

COACH G STATS   108

ACKNOWLEDGMENTS

A special thank you to my wife, Kimberlynn, who has always been my biggest cheerleader. She is forever pushing me to be better, to dream big, and never settle for anything. Our journey together has made me grow and mature both mentally and emotionally. I thank you for all that you are and all that you inspire me to be. Thank you for creating the AP's (Accountability Partners), our collection of visionary friends who help us continue to dream and be.

To Mr. McGowen, you see things in me that I can only dream of being one day, but our conversations continue to ignite the desire in me to continue to pursue my destiny. I appreciate your love for sports and your heart for what is right and true. I am honored to call you a friend and a mentor.

Coach P, you have always been the greatest inspiration to me as a coach and a friend. Your wisdom never ceases to amaze me. Your constant acknowledgment of my talents and abilities keeps me motivated and striving for excellence. Thank you for always believing in me and freely providing me with all your wealth of knowledge to get through all my adventurous endeavors. I am forever grateful.

To my Principal, Dr. Phyllis Cormier. Thank you for allowing me to be me, the teacher, and the coach. You have no hesitation in placing me in the right positions to use my talents. Additionally, thank you for providing me the opportunities to grow in our profession and my coaching. I am so grateful and have such high regard for you, as a person and as my boss.

Lastly, I want to thank my Lord and Savior, Jesus Christ, for my life's journey. I am anchored in my faith, and I seek your counsel freely. I know whose I am and why I am still here. Thank you for every person you continuously place in my life to grow me and keep me focused on you and your word. As an educator, I pride myself on doing your work to help others because with every life I touch, the more blessings I seem to continuously receive, and I am grateful for them all.

PRE-GAME

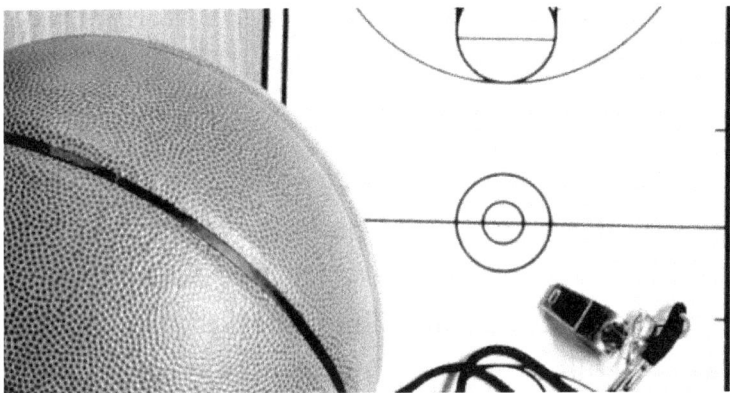

Imagine going off to college and looking forward to the day when you can put that degree to work. I remember the exhilarating feeling like yesterday. I was excited, nervous, and anxious all at once as I crossed the stage in my cap and gown. I had the degree, but I could not utilize the accolade yet. I was honored to have been chosen as the new head basketball coach and assistant volleyball coach for a middle school program. After meeting with the campus coordinator and Principal, I was given the keys to the campus. This is the moment where reality began to set in. Worry began to run a full-court press in my mind. What is my salary; will it be enough to take care of myself, being completely on my own in a new city? Did I accept the offer too soon? Is there other paperwork for me to sign? Am I ready to lead these student-athletes?

Of course, the following week, I was given instructions on the next steps, remember this is 1994, and emails were not popular; so, you had to make a point to find the right person to ask the questions and get the phone number of whom to contact. Consequently, it all worked out. I was fortunate to have coaches that treated me like family and made sure I did what was expected of me to exceed the expectations for my position. During this time, I realized that people are your greatest resources in this profession. Coaches have a camaraderie that provides a sense of belonging like nothing else.

It is with great hope that this book will fulfill its purpose, to assist coaches in creating an environment conducive to learning and performance achievement. Additionally, being a guide to developing a successful athletic program that produces exceptional student-athletes who inspire positive and productive men and women of today's society. Consequently, generating transformational coaches who will inspire other coaches to do more than just coach.

My reason for writing this book is simple. It is a resource for those new to the coaching game or those currently coaching but who have not completely figured out what it takes to build and sustain a great program. I often felt I was missing key elements to be a successful coach, especially when my record did not meet the school's expectations.

Numbers in my program dropped from one season to the other, and this was very frustrating, especially because I did not know why. I have since learned that there are many reasons that program numbers will drop. The dislike of the school and what the school is not providing academically or athletically is a major consideration. The economy or major disasters and life situations are a few thoughts for you to ponder. How arrogant of me to think I was solely responsible for my program's numbers. I was accountable, but there are contributing factors beyond my reach.

I am by no means a Pat Summit or Geno Auriemma, although they are my mentors, but I strive in every way to be a coach that does more than just coach student-athletes. I want to provide something intangible, something so imperative that everyone wants to learn and become a part of. I have learned so much in my 28 years of teaching and coaching, and it is time to share with my colleagues.

CHAPTER I
JUMP BALL

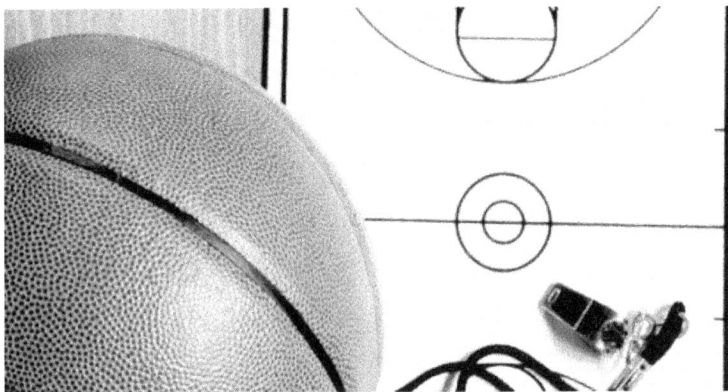

Huddle Up! I am Coach G. I have been a coach for over 28 years. This year, I just accepted a head coaching position for a local high school in Houston, TX. I am more prepared and more at peace with this transition than any I have had before. Do you wish to know why? Experience, education, and the willingness to follow my passion, no matter what. I train athletes. I mentor students and teachers. I am never afraid to step out of my comfort zone if it continues to lead me to my destiny and grow. I want that for every coach out there! I am here to show the plays that have prepared me.

I have been in the game long enough to know there is an automatic expectation that coaches know everything and make things happen, no matter the circumstance. Honestly, we are competitors; we are built to overcome obstacles. We will bust our asses to figure it out. I have gotten the job and the keys in one day. Some wear this experience as a badge of honor; however, it is not the correct way to transition to a new position or a new school.

My true purpose for writing this book is to provide a checklist to coaches who are new to the profession. Coaches just want to ensure they provide the best experience for their staff and student-athletes, on and off the court. Furthermore, it can make for a less stressful situation in addition to the responsibilities of the job itself.

GAME PLAN

Huddle Up! will assist coaches with creating an environment that is conducive for learning, performance, and achievement, that incorporates every aspect of an individual's existence, and improves personal skill development. This playbook will identify the most important areas to building a successful basketball program. We cover everything from the transformational leadership coaching style to the formation of exceptional student-athletes.

TRANSFORMATIONAL COACH

Transformational coaches are a necessity in the athletic realm on every level. This type of coach creates a real-world experience for their athletes. They view athletics as an opportunity to inspire and transform their athletes into student-athletes. Student-athletes experience athletics from many perspectives. For many, sports provide and implement discipline, structure, and organization. The locker room is a place to experience love, family, and the appreciation of others and oneself. As a transformational leader, I aspire to use my chosen profession to transform the lives of all student-athletes. There must be a vision bigger than statistics and wins to be a transformational coach. A philosophy that incorporates every aspect of the program from the coaching staff to the student–athletes, the school district, and the community. An awareness of the product and an analysis of what it takes to sustain and grow it is vital to creating a successful program. A transformational coach understands the importance of adhering to the code of ethics, the rules and regulations of the state and school district, and the significant impact non-adherence could have on a coach's program.

I consider myself a transformational coach. Like any coach, I always coach to win. However, I have learned over time that sometimes we gain so much more when we lose. Basketball, for me, is a way of learning life, as many sports are. You experience many highs and lows. You are challenged daily, and every day that you are, you have to do better, be better, and work harder. Over time it literally becomes a way of life outside of the sport. Success is the only thing. Doing well at being a parent, a sibling, a friend, and a teacher is a rite of passage.

I strive to develop relationships that go beyond basketball with every team I coach. Once the season is over, I continue to encourage my players to be the best at the game of life. Unfortunately, not every student-athlete makes it to the pros. That does not mean they cannot be a pro at whatever the game of life throws at them. As a coach for the Houston Lady Nets, I received great feedback from the community. My coaching style was what the parents and staff felt the girls needed. Often training sessions were not just about basketball; they were moments to uplift broken spirits, to pass on a new perspective about life, or just have someone willing to listen. Being with the Houston Lady Nets program gave me a sense of helping the community, not just coaching basketball.

STUDENT-ATHLETE

It is important to understand the weight student-athletes carry. They are maturing in all areas of their life while striving to exceed expectations. To be a student-athlete, one must be willing to go beyond the boundaries of personal achievement. The ability to work when no one else is working or looking. Possessing the power to work with others who want exactly what you want and are willing to do whatever is necessary to acquire the all-American and other top player awards within the legal limits, of course. The ability to work with others and learn from others, be scrutinized by others, and sometimes be led by others whose vision does not align with yours. Balancing all these responsibilities can be difficult and make the public question a player's dedication. This can trickle down to the players themselves. There is a way to live in this crazy world we call sports and make every moment meaningful and your journey an enjoyable one.

First, let's become a student-athlete. Create more than just a player's mentality but a mentality that goes beyond being just a player. It is important that my student-athletes work on building skill sets, strengthening their bodies, conditioning their minds, and studying strategies to be great players. However, to be successful and perform according to the expectations of the program, they must implement methods of mental training and psychological development to deal with the behaviors and emotional states of mind that will occur because of the requirements to excel and be the best. Therefore, creating methods for managing stress, anxiety, self-doubt, lack of confidence, and lack of motivation creates better sports performance, enhances self-direction, career advancement, and personal/team success in sports and other areas of their lives.

ACTION PLAN

Setting goals can give us a clear vision of where we are and where we would like to be, individually and collectively. Having a system for stress management can alleviate behavioral problems and breakdowns in team collaboration and performance. Incorporating methods/skills for communication does assist with providing a climate where everyone has a voice. Providing team cohesion methods helps develop skills and self-awareness and creates the needed environment to improve performance. Implementing plans of action, inclusive of professional development for coaches, community outreach with players, and the school can profoundly impact one's program. As an educator, I consistently motivate my students to be their best. It starts with setting goals. For example, waking up every day and making up their bed. Completing an assignment or arriving to school on time. It is rewarding to see how setting these simple goals can change their vision. As a coach, I teach my student-athletes that it is ok to make mistakes as long as we recover, move on, and improve our work ethic. As a leader, I communicate with my staff, make it we, not me, and allow them to have a voice and a say.

In conclusion, the purpose for coaching any sport is always bigger than the sport itself. The experiences and knowledge gained through that sport plant the seeds that provide for the growth and development of exceptional student-athletes who become transformational leaders of the future.

CHAPTER II
PHILOSOPHY OF COACHING ATHLETICS

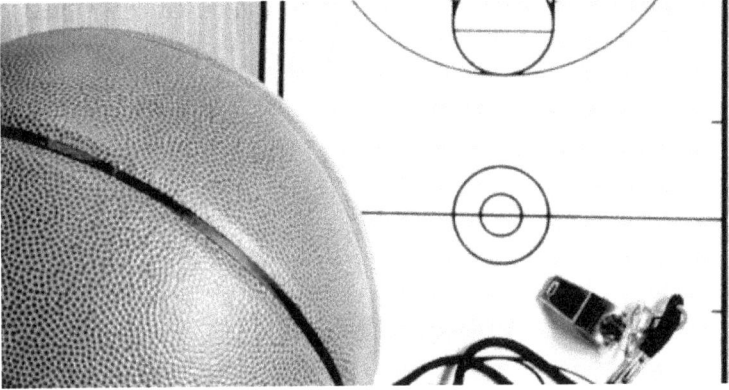

MISSION STATEMENT

To approach the game as one approaches life, anticipating the future, setting goals every step of the way, and seeking and creating opportunities for success.

Everyone wants to succeed in life, but it often seems impossible. The approach is a means to simplify and experience the realities of life so that success is inevitable by implementing the necessary tools to create a portfolio of the journey and its challenges, with solutions that provide clear explanations of its rewards. One must believe and understand the importance of education and what it means to achieve academic excellence. In the same respect, as individuals, we acknowledge the significance of being responsible for our every action and behavior. Through the game of basketball, we strive to represent and uphold these truths, whether winning or losing; therefore, it never feels like failure, only success.

VISION STATEMENT:

To be the defining role models of success.

There is always a question of who exemplifies a great role model. A professional athlete? An actor or entertainer? The president? Oprah Winfrey? My response is always the same. Anyone can be a role model: you must be willing to do the right things, possess the right attitude, be a servant, and be willing to humble yourself and speak up for what you believe in. I challenge my athletes to be role models daily, no matter what role they may be playing, because someone is always watching.

Our challenges are so often other people's solutions to their problems or circumstances.

At one point in my career, my Director was persistent in firmly encouraging me to take the head position for the Lady Hurricanes. The Lady Hurricanes had a reputation of being combative, being tardy, and not adhering to the request of their coaches. I was coaching the men's team, and we had great success the past few years. So, this brought about the discussion. I understood that as a director, you want all your programs to be successful, so with a little apprehension but a bit of excitement for the challenge, I embraced the opportunity. Yes, changes happened, and the women's program received academic honors and two seasons of conference finals!

I approached the challenge with my truth to create an open door of communication, a sense of self-worth, a sense of belonging, and a vision of personal success, not just on the court success.

In an article written by Molly Fletcher, a keynote speaker and author, she addressed "The 5 Core Values Behind Pat Summit is Legendary

Leadership." One of those five core values, Build Trust Through Fairness, revealed what I honestly tried to implement with my players. She states that the single most important principle of teaching is, "They don't care how much you know unless they know how much you care." With this philosophy in mind, we have been the top seed for the last two semesters and made it to the Championship game both times. We are still waiting for the title, but we have made great strides in being the role models our campus expects us to be.

CORE VALUES

Core Values are your personal beliefs that shape who you are. Your core values determine your responses to situations, your feelings to issues and problems that arise, and how you respond in those instances. It is important to know who you are and to understand why you are who you are. Transparency is so much easier when you understand your core values. As a transformational coach, you are not afraid to say where you come from, what you have experienced, and how it made you feel. These things help build trust and create a safe space for you and your student-athletes.

1. TO FIND THE GOOD IN EVERYONE AND NURTURE IT.

There is something unique about every individual. Those who possess it often go unnoticed, but others see it. When it comes to developing chemistry within your team members, it is essential that some form of connection brings about conversation. This connection links a player's ability to motivate and build lasting relationships. For example, what are their dreams and goals outside of basketball? What kind of life would they like to live? What does happiness look like to you? What do you enjoy? Communication and conversation outside the scope of the game is so instrumental to understanding your players. You begin to see them as individuals with life goals and situations just like you, not just one of your players in a jersey.

2. TO BE WILLING TO ALWAYS BETTER THEIR BEST.

We as human beings tend to get complacent when things are going well and we are reaching new heights. Therefore, doing more than the minimum is often a struggle. I want to always instill in my athletes that there is always someone better, someone working harder. Let that be you.

3. LET FEAR PROPEL YOU, NOT STOP YOU.

In the route to success, fear is the one thing that stops one from fulfilling his or her destiny. The fear of the unknown. The fear of family/ friend disconnect. The fear of being successful. The fear of failure. I feel it is necessary to incorporate it as a core value because it is one of those primary reasons we often fail to reach our fullest potential.

Marianne Williamson's poem about fear says it best: "Our deepest fear is not that we are inadequate. Our deepest fear is that we are powerful beyond measure. It is our light, not our darkness, that frightens us."

The leadership styles that I will implement to work with athletes and coaches today will be cooperative and transformational. I prefer to use sports as a tool for life's lessons. Many situations occur when performing, preparing or living life as an athlete that are reflective of life's experiences. "Coaches who adopt the cooperative style focus on teaching. This includes teaching not only technical and tactical skills but life-skills as well" (Martens 2004, p.29). I have always admired Phil Jackson's coaching style and his approach that everyone on the team should participate in play, not just those one or two-star players. I am not afraid to sacrifice winning for that teachable moment or that moment that can change the way an athlete or coach feels at that moment. Through those special moments, teams may thrive and get a clear vision of our mission.

Transformational leadership is the ability to create and transform. As a coach, I relish the individual achievements of my players. It is very rewarding to see my team grow and mature into great leaders today. Transformational leaders strive to help followers become leaders themselves. Therefore, when I coach, I want to influence my players, coaches, and everyone who contributes to my program. I want my mission and vision to be clear and precise, with no questions of what our program is completely about...Athletes First, Winning Second!

CHAPTER III
BEYOND THE COURT

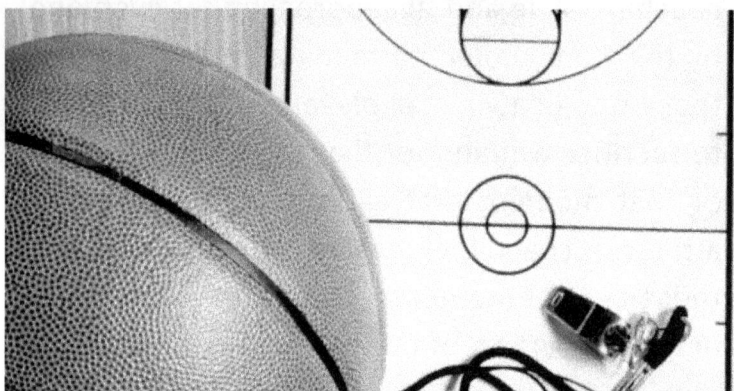

The best way to teach the game is to have as much knowledge about the game as possible. Education is my second love. I received my Master of Education in Coaching and Athletic Administration from Concordia University. My research delivers my passion for the health of all students, not just the athletes. The idea of being a transformational leader is looking at every aspect of the population being led. In consideration of the high rates of obesity, because of inactivity and the emphasis on academics and testing, versus the physical welfare of our youth, drives this research study.

Research has proven that by incorporating physical activity into the academic arena, brain activity increases and enhances learning.

The research considers the question of, is there an improvement in academic performance when high school students participate in moderate to vigorous physical activity during a school semester in the low-income areas in Houston, Texas? Times have changed where participating in physical activities is often not a priority for parents. It tends to be quite costly and time-consuming. However, when we consider our lower-income areas, this population is more prone to encourage participation in hopes of an athletic opportunity for college. Consequently, we find that these students begin to perform well academically because of their vision of a possible athletic scholarship. If we refocus the vision and use that physical activity with academic challenges, it is possible to improve the overall academic performance for all students and decrease the obesity population.

Incorporating *Huddle Up* in your game plan ensures ideas are provoked and processes for change can occur. Improvement in academic and athletic performance is the focus.

When considering a research question, the idea of physical activity and academic performance came to mind. The academic achievements of high school students are constantly changing from year to year. With the world's economic problems, it is of utmost importance that the educational system makes the necessary adjustments to ensure student success. However, in the classrooms, teachers and administrators find it more of a challenge to get students engaged and excited about learning. Academic success or achievement is a necessary component to a comfortable future. Creating an environment where students are engaged physically and mentally has become a new way of teaching for some.

There are many studies about the importance of physical activity and its role in assisting students with learning. However, athletics prove this every day. Students who participate in sports are more likely to perform better in classes to continue to play their chosen sport; no pass, no play rule is real in Texas. For example, I had a student who loved playing football, but due to his consistent misbehavior in classes and at home, he was placed in a behavioral management class with no more than seven students. I remember him asking, "What would it take for me to play football?" My response was, "Improve your behavior so that you can be in regular classes and speak with the coach about what he needs from you to play." Within three weeks' time, his behavior made a 180-degree turn. He was removed from the class and into regular classes and became part of the football team. My soul was elated. This is an example of behavior change. However, I have witnessed students have great grades during their sports season, and grades drop once the season is over. No more motivation, no one holding them accountable. However, a transformational coach will always expect success on and off the court, in-season, or out of season. Because the individual student-athlete is more than just a student-athlete, they are a young man or woman trying to make something of themselves and have an impact on the future of this world.

There are also many studies about overweight and obese kids. As stated in an active living research brief, one in three children in the United States is overweight or obese. Obese youth have an elevated risk for health problems like heart disease, type 2 diabetes, high blood pressure, unhealthy blood cholesterol patterns, and other health risks related to cardiovascular disease. "Obesity can also have serious ramifications for kids' cognitive development and affect school attendance" (Castelli, 2015 p. 1).

Therefore, for this research study, the focus question will be: Is there an improvement in academic performance when high school students participate in moderate to vigorous physical activity during a school semester in the low-income areas in Houston, Texas? To define low-income areas concerning schools, for example, most of the schools in the Houston area are Title 1 schools which require extra funding from the state to ensure student achievement. Moderate to vigorous physical activity has a means to an end that could be two-fold in assisting students in living more productive and healthier lives, both physically and intellectually.

STATEMENT OF THE PROBLEM

Is there an improvement in academic performance when high school students participate in moderate to vigorous physical activity during a school semester in the low-income areas in Houston, Texas? The irony that surrounds the population of high school students that grow up in low-income areas revolve around one thing: athletic ability. If they are good at sports, the likelihood of academic success is heightened because of their desire to use their physical ability to remove themselves and their families from poverty. But, what about the students who are incapable of achieving athletic prowess or success academically? The duty of a school district is to ensure all students graduate, despite their economic circumstances. Therefore, will incorporating a regular moderate to vigorous physical activity class or program for students to engage in on a consistent basis improve their desire to perform better in academics?

Having the opportunity to teach in a low-income area provided a clear vision of what life was truly about for them. Acquiring an education was important because it was expected. However, the achievement often seemed very daunting for some. Being involved with activities and sports gave them a sense of belonging, in addition to having someone who cared and would hold them accountable. As a coach, it is important to believe in all students and have a desire for them to succeed. When dealing with their issues, I found myself wanting to know more and do more. With this research, the hope is that it proves that by participating in moderate to vigorous physical activity low-income high school students can make improvements in their academic performance.

As indicated in the research introduction by Castelli, both childhood obesity and poor academic performance tend to be clustered in schools with a high percentage of lower-income, minority students, creating a student health issue that is especially problematic in those communities (p.1). This is very evident in the Houston metro area because most of the schools' populations are minority and low-income. The focus at this point is to generate revenue for those schools to provide those students with the necessary physical activities inside and outside of the classrooms to negate this epidemic. Incorporating various forms of moderate to vigorous physical activities for students to participate in on a regular basis will generate better academic performance, as we will demonstrate, and healthier communities.

The state of Texas uses the Fitness Gram program by The Cooper Institute to assess students' levels of fitness in their physical education classes in schools. The health-related fitness components are assessed: aerobic capacity, muscular endurance, muscular strength, flexibility, and body composition. The Fitness Gram uses the pacer, one-mile, curl-ups, push-ups, and BMI tests to get an idea of the level of fitness students are currently in on a yearly basis. However, it does not provide any information on how the students' fitness level affects their academic performance; it is a test of physical fitness, not mental fitness.

In 2010, Houston ISD took part in a study titled, *Correlational and Predictive Analysis of Obesity on Student Achievement Using*

HISD Fitness Gram Results, 2008-2009. The study assumes that health is correlated with academic achievement, and those efforts to combat obesity are reflected in school health and physical education programs (Holmes, 2010, pg. 1). The interesting factors were in the economic status and ethnicity. The study sample was taken from economically disadvantaged (at-risk) students and those designated as special education program participants. "With their findings, considering the BMI factor specifically in relation to academic performance: Higher scores in reading, math, language, and science among Asian, African American, Hispanic and White students were found to be significantly correlated with lower BMIs. Moreover, students with above-average math and reading scores were more likely not to experience obesity. These results are relevant since brain research documents "cognitive development occurs in tandem" with physical activity" (CDC, 2010, p.13).

To improve obesity, there must be a physically motivated movement to engage students to desire to be more physically active. Moderate to vigorous physical activity is not just standing up and taking a break but increasing the heart rate, stimulating the energy in the brain, and providing the body with movement that generates a constant desire for a motion— for example, dancing for 1 minute with your arms going above your head and your feet doing a variety of steps coming off the floor interchangeably or jogging in place or skipping around the room. If students are outside, team games like tag and relay races not only get their bodies moving but allow their minds to think and strategize how to win critically. With that being stated, per Trost and Va Der Mars, it is critical that school districts build sustainable and effective physical education programs by implementing population-based strategies and interventions. This is particularly critical since "decreasing time in physical education does not significantly improve academic performance" (2009, p.62).

REVIEW OF THE LITERATURE

However, there were studies outside of the previously mentioned Fitness gram study in 2010, which addressed the issue of the implementation of community-based programs that would assist with the incorporation of more physical activity. For example, the CATCH El Paso program has generated significant interest in "living healthy" lifestyles for families through more physical activity. The CATCH (Coordinated Approach to Child Health) program is a comprehensive and fun approach to Whole Child Health that addresses physical activity, nutrition, stress reduction, vaping, prevention, and more.

It is not surprising that adding intensive community involvement to a school-based program leads to strong results in reducing childhood obesity. Studies of children's eating habits show that the environment out of school—at home and in the broader community—matters as much or more than the school environment. A community-school partnership ensures that a child's environment supports healthy living at school and beyond school. The El Paso format ensures that families and community members participate in modeling and encouraging healthy choices for children (Arons, 2011. p. 32). This approach can help the Houston area youth create an outside-in approach to improving academic performance through a physical activity community-based approach.

In a study by Russel Atkinson, *Does Physical Activity Improve Academic Performance*, he added a daily vigorous physical activity into the curriculum during a semester with 11th-grade students who were experiencing a lack of academic success. Students recorded very positive improvements in daily attendance, overall credit accumulation, and perhaps most impressively, a massive decline in the number of days of suspension. "We became convinced that the academic performance of the entire school would improve with increased physical activity" (Atkinson, 2010, pg. 22). In addition to Atkinson's study, an EDUFIT study was done to analyze the effects of an intervention focused on increasing the time and intensity of Physical Education on adolescents' cognitive performance and academic performance. Here the results revealed that an increase in the intensity of the physical education sessions might play a role in the positive effects of physical activity and academic success (Ardoy, 2014, p.52). Consequently, providing mental and physical health benefits to today's youth from a variety of socio-economic backgrounds. Considering the research, it is apparent that moderate to vigorous physical activity impacts academic performance. Studies are constantly being done to prove its need and will heed the removal of physical education at any level.

A sample of senior-level students will be taken from several of the district's high schools to on the growing evidence of physical activity and academic performance from a cognitive research perspective. This study will address the distinction of the impact of the intensity or level of physical activity and its effect on academic performance for low-income students in the Houston Independent School District. Low income, for this study, is defined as children living in families of four or more with a household income below $48,016. This study is reliable because the primary data source that will be used is required by the school district.

PROFESSIONAL IMPLICATIONS

The findings in this study support a concern of not just the physical health of our youth but the academic success of our youth. When considering ways to improve academic performance for all populations, physical activity of some kind is a necessary tool. As previous research shows, regular participation in physical activity and higher levels of physical fitness have been linked to improved academic performance and brain functions, such as attention and memory. These brain functions are the foundation for learning (Castelli, 2015).

As studies advance to specific populations, the evidence will show the need for more moderate to vigorous physical activity for school-aged children and youth. Participating in physical activity is necessary for everyone, regardless of age. However, when we look at the future, it is not just a necessity. Physical activity needs to be a constant and expected fixture in every classroom and curriculum.

Although this study was specific to the Houston ISD low-income population of students, other areas of the state can benefit from this study and be considered a broader representation sample for this study. Furthermore, this study can benefit many other areas of the United States who deal with this socio-economic population of students. As the researcher, it would be enlightening to see the responses from various geographical areas, like the EDUFIT Study, which took place in Spain. In conclusion, this research can be a beneficial tool for today's coaches by generating a more physically active sector of youth that will bring about a better understanding of sports performance.

CHAPTER IV
ETHICS AND SPORTSMANSHIP

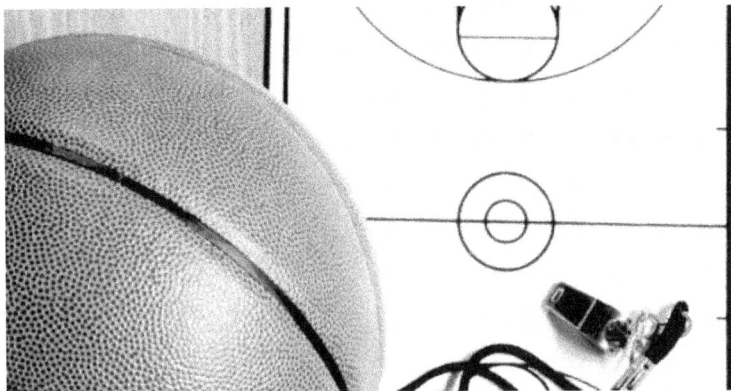

Coaches and athletic administrators are leaders and models for good sportsmanship and ethical behavior. They are responsible for upholding the codes of conduct, standards of behavior, and integrity of all members of the program, including the coaches, support staff, and student-athletes. For this reason, those who lead and set the example for others must clearly understand the virtues and civic responsibilities that they are to uphold. *The Ten Christian Virtues and Civic Responsibilities of Coaches and Administrators as Leaders of Sport in the 21st Century* serves as a guideline for the men and women who teach, coach, and lead. Three of the Christian virtues and civic responsibility that are particularly important for coaches and leaders in sports are serving, humble, and enthusiastic.

SERVING

Service is a word that can have many meanings. However, in every definition, it relates to someone doing something for someone else. The most common definition is the performance of duties or services for another person or organization. Greenleaf's explanation of service as a leadership position: Servant leadership begins with the notion that one wants to serve others. The servant–leader transforms his or her thought process to align with the needs of others rather than with personal desires. The servant–leader must change his/her thinking from "what is it that I want?" to "what is it that is needed?" Further, servant leaders perceive their role from the perspective of what impact their actions have on others (Greenleaf, 2002). (Lumpkin, Stoll, & Beller, 2012 Pg. 43)

Being of service to others is a quality that all coaches should embrace. It is a coach's duty to serve their athletes in a way that helps them to become more than they can ever imagine. To consistently challenge them to be women and men of character and see their lives through a window bigger than the sport they play. As a coach of service, the development of the physicality of their athletes is important, as well as the psychological development of those athletes as human beings and contributors to today's society.

HUMBLE

Humble is having or showing a modest or low estimate of one's importance. A great example of being humble is Coach John Wooden. Coach Wooden never wanted special privileges. Frank Arnold, a former assistant coach of Coach Wooden, recalled the time when he and Coach Wooden got in line to register for the National Association of Basketball Coaches at the Final Four on an occasion when Coach Wooden's Bruins were there to play their eighth national championship.

Coach Arnold states, "The line was enormous, and here is John Wooden at the back of the line when we were a participant in the tournament. People kept telling him, 'Coach, go to the front of the line, pay your dues, and get out of here.' He would not do that. We stood in that doggone line for an hour and a half to pay our twenty-dollar dues. We could have gone to the front, but he wouldn't. He wanted to be an ordinary guy, but he certainly was not an ordinary guy" (ACE Blog, 2016).

In his book, *Season of Life*, Joe Ehrmann creates an amazing example of a man who takes the experiences of his life and generates an amazing picture of the truth about what sports and coaching are about. For the coaches of today, it is crucial for them to see past the scoreboard and see their games as tools to provide an experience for the future of their athletes.

Ehrmann's mission for his boys at Gilman-Building Men for Others Program states, "Being a man means emphasizing relationships and having a cause bigger than yourself. It means accepting responsibility and leading courageously" (Marx, J. 2003). Therefore, today's coaches should focus more on creating lasting relationships with their athletes and transforming programs that are truly based on a defined philosophy and mission.

ENTHUSIASM

Enthusiasm, according to Merriam-Webster, is defined as a strong excitement about something or a strong feeling of active interest in something that you like or enjoy.

A great example of enthusiasm (passion) is Kim Mulky, former Head Coach for the Baylor University Women's Basketball team, now Head Coach of Louisiana State University Women's Basketball program. Her enthusiasm for the game is so vividly evident in everything she does for Women's basketball.

She is the first person in NCAA Women's basketball history to win a national championship as a player, assistant coach, and head coach. Her resiliency in what she believes and desires for her program and others is undeniably praiseworthy and completely contagious. She believes in a community effort. The people who make up the university/high school community play a major role in building quality programs. Having community support in the stands at games and developing a belief in the student-athletes and their coaches is like having an extra player that helps to create a great program.

When considering the experts in the field of sports, those coaches that are the most successful possess a passion for the sport they coach, but the enthusiasm is what comes from the responses they receive from their athletes. John Wooden states, "Leaders must always generate enthusiasm if they wish to bring out the best in themselves and others." Great coaches should have a passion for what they do. Great coaches should believe in their mission and goals and get excited about every single step being made to achieve those goals. Enthusiasm cannot be taught. It should just be in you; it is an internal virtue.

The coaches that pride themselves on being humble, enthusiastic, and are willing to serve will find great meaning and appreciation to the benefits that come. These qualities are me. I am a very humble person. I will never forget the dark moments when basketball was my beacon of hope. I aim to share that light with every student–athlete that sits on my bleachers. Our transparent communication bonds us on and off the court.

When I watch coaches like Kim Mulkey, Pat Summit, and Dawn Staley, I see myself. I find great satisfaction in helping not just student–athletes but anyone who wants to pursue their passion or a dream. Moreover, the greatest pleasure of becoming an educator and coach was that I get to experience these qualities every day. It is what I do. Therefore, going to work is not a job; it is a daily adventure.

CHAPTER V
LEGAL ASPECTS AND CONSIDERATIONS

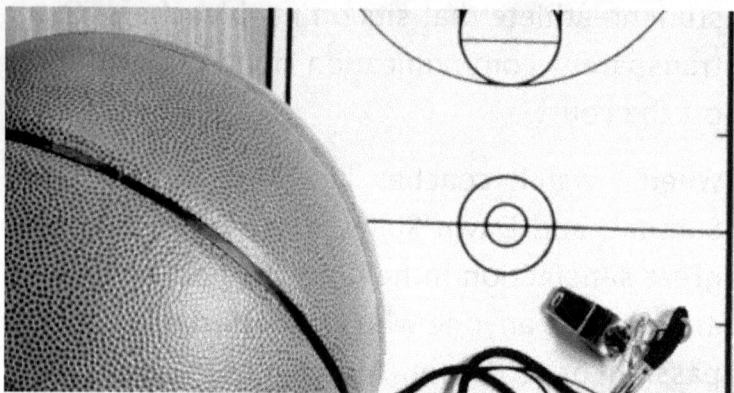

As a coach, one must consider the legal aspects that come with the job of managing middle school to high school-aged students. Considerations from who is supervising to the location of supervision, to the accommodations being used, equipment, language used, and the list of processes and procedures, per the district, to be followed. As a coach or athletic administrator, it is important to know who is working with athletes, parents, or school districts for the safety and protection of the students. Nonetheless, for the image and integrity of the programs that represent those entities as well.

By ensuring that every district has a risk management plan, legal aspects and considerations can be addressed accordingly or even prevented. A risk management plan, or RMP, helps identify the risks, determine the necessary areas in which these risks may or will affect, create specific methods to reduce those risks from occurring, and a means of management within those occurrences. Visit the UIL website to see what rules apply to your region or state.

The Legal Duties of Athletic Personnel are important to the functionalityof athletic programs. These duties provide general guidelines to the structure of programs and how coaches, staff, and administrators should perform. Additionally, these duties are guidelines to prevent legal implications and the insurance of proper management, supervision, training, and coaching of student-athletes. The two legal duties that will be clarified are the duty to supervise and the duty to instruct properly.

DUTY TO SUPERVISE

A coach must be physically present, provide supervision, control players' impulsive behavior, provide competent instruction, structure practices that are appropriate for the age and maturity of players, prevent foreseeable injuries, and respond to injury or trauma in an approved manner. Supervision requires diligence and knowledge of issues that are likely to occur and the ability to ensure procedures are taken to prevent those occurrences. For example, physical education classes tend to be quite large in middle schools. Proper supervision is critical to preventing injuries when overseeing large group activities. Maintain a reasonable coach–to–student ratio. In high schools, when competing in high–risk activities, such as wrestling and gymnastics, supervision and safety precautions must be clearly defined.

Athletic administrators' supervisory duties consider the coaching staff's ability and performance regarding their required responsibilities and management of student-athletes. Additionally, the appropriateness of behavior of spectators at contests, the facilities in which student–athletes use and perform, the conditions of the weather, and the necessary steps to take when it is too dangerous for competition to engage or continue.

The situation in which the duty of supervision is trying to avoid or correct is negligence on behalf of the coaches, administration, and staff. Accidents can and will happen, but they are less likely with proper supervision. By creating an environment conducive to safe participation and free from any form of danger, legalities of negligence can be prevented.

Programs that do not consider the number of students participating in physical education classes are failing to comply with the duty of supervision. A gym with 120 students, two certified teachers, and one aide is not adequate supervision, and neither is a gym with one certified teacher/coach and 50 students. The changes that would need to be made would be like a secondary classroom setting -- a minimum 35 to 1 ratio or another certified teacher/coach trained to handle the situations that may occur. According to the Texas education code, there is a regulation regarding the class size limit for PE. TEC §25.114 requires the implementation of PE curriculum, to the extent practicable, utilizing student/teacher ratios that are small enough to ensure the safety of students. If the school district establishes a student/teacher ratio greater than 45 to 1 in a PE class, the district shall specifically identify the way the safety of the students will be maintained (Texas Education Agency, 2015).

Considering the aforementioned regulation, some ideas to consider would be providing professional development to coaches to assist with handling large groups and understanding the risks of lack of proper supervision. Creating team leaders in the gym can help with supervision. In addition, providing students the opportunity to help set up equipment, be line leaders for attendance, and post class rules in specific areas to remind students of daily expectations can greatly assist with adhering to the duty to supervise.

DUTY TO INSTRUCT PROPERLY

The duty to instruct properly involves consideration and understanding of the growth and development of the human body, not about which student-athlete can do the skill the best and the focus on winning. Proper instruction begins with proper and appropriate training of a specific sport or entity. The deliverance of that training is the key to the progression and achievement of each individual student-athlete. For example, placing a coach in a position of a sport that he or she is not familiar with poses a huge risk to the student-athlete and the program.

The purpose of the duty to instruct properly is to ensure proper progression of the knowledge and skill of a sports' techniques, application, and risks. Knowing the risks of sports, coaches should make a point to learn the necessary skills sets, training techniques, performance measurements, and fundamentals.

A long-term commitment to physical literacy and proper training to improve athleticism and sports-skill development is vital for optimal athletic potential. Proper training and athletic development can be time-consuming. Moreover, a paradigm shift needs to occur regarding the pace and process of athletic development (Meadors, p. 6).

When considering this duty, it is important to consider the defenses against negligence, inherent risks, and negligence risks. Coaches have a duty to negate these risks with proper instruction, proper training, and consistent awareness of those things that may cause harm to student-athletes. For example, "Primary assumption of risk is presumed when an individual has voluntarily participated in an activity that involves inherent or well-known risks" (Coton & Wolohan, 2013, p.79). However, as a coach with knowledge of these risks, it is in their best interest to address, train, and prepare student-athletes for these risks. Likewise, administrators must provide opportunities for coaches to be trained on how to instruct, demonstrate, and identify these risks.

Understanding the importance of supervision and instruction should be a well-developed coaching philosophy. Unfortunately, it is often the reason for many injuries, accidents, and administrative infractions. Athletics is a place where injuries will occur. However, it is up to the coaches to ensure that it was just an assumption of risk injury and not negligence on the coaches and administration. Proper education and professional development are instrumental for coaches to understand the importance of proper instruction.

I instruct as though my athletes are blank canvases that have never seen a gym. I make sure instructions are clear and concise and provide examples and key terminology to ensure understanding and comprehension for everyone. There is a saying that says, "Great teachers make great coaches." For example, during pre-season, it is a perfect time to explain to student-athletes why we must train, the importance of nutrition, and the benefits of knowing the rules and language of your sport. Additionally, the reason we have only 5 minutes to get dressed and get out of the locker room is to prevent horseplay, creating a focus on why we are here instead of issues on social media.

Lastly, always have a timed agenda for practices, and share it with your athletes prior to the next practice. This way, everyone is aware of their expectations and where they are to be. Taking the time to include everyone in daily practices can greatly assist in preventing injuries, accidents, and administrative infractions. Communication is the key!

CHAPTER VI
PROGRAM DEVELOPMENT

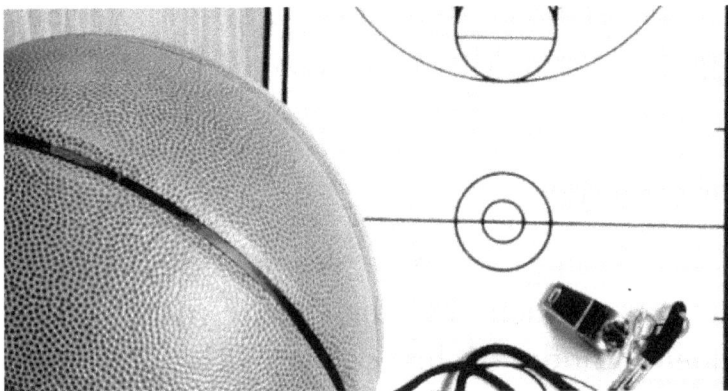

A successful program is well organized and structured. The program is considerate of all factors, from the requirements of the school district to the needs of the community. Programs thrive when their nucleus is the welfare of the student–athletes in respect to their achievements outside of the program, success in the classroom, and their future careers. All these things must be considered. The growth and expertise of the staff and assistants must be reflective of the head coach's vision and mission of the program. Successful programs are not just about wins and losses but the ultimate growth and development of positive and productive young men and women leaders for today's society. Consequently, demonstrating the type of program that produces great student-athletes is the pride of the school district and community.

ORGANIZATION

The organization of a program starts with communication by the head coach. The identification of his or her vision for the program and the necessary factors that will ensure that vision is met. Communicating their vision and expectations to the athletes, parents, and coaches creates a relationship that can ensure a community-wide effort in a successful program.

The use of technology makes communication easier. Playbooks, master schedules, posting schedules, and keeping parents informed about the happenings of the program can be at everyone's immediate access. For example, HUDL is a very good program that can aid in all those areas. The return to campus after the COVID shutdown required some additional innovation. To accommodate COVID gathering restrictions and parents' schedules, I utilized popular video meeting software to keep everyone informed and involved.

Furthermore, the Student Handbook, Coaches Manual, and the Parent Athletic Handbook are resources that head coaches must provide for the athletes, parents, and coaches before beginning the season. These items outline the vision and mission of the program, the expectation of the player, parents, and coaches, and specific responsibilities, rules, and regulations about game day routines and behavior expectations for all. The head coach must communicate effectively and often to negate any unforeseen situations. Team, parent, and coaches' meetings are very important to ensure that everyone is on the same page and aware of their roles within the program. More specifically, identifying the responsibilities for coaches, trainers, and support staff. The dictation of responsibilities helps with the consistent and efficient flow of the program, creating a positive and more productive environment that everyone enjoys.

Lastly, one key element that is important to a head coach's organization and can strategically outline the entire season is a master calendar. This calendar provides a clear picture of the overall season and the happenings of the program, including but not limited to games, practices, tournaments, meetings, and outside events like fundraising. The master calendar can be beneficial in assisting parents with planning doctors' appointments and vacations for their children without the concern of missing practices or games.

TEAM PRACTICE

Team practice sessions must be well organized, detailed, and specific. A daily agenda identifying the skills to be covered must be listed. It is beneficial to the success of the program that practices encompass areas of tactile and technical drills, strength and conditioning, position specific and team drills. It is important to consider the duration of the drills and the rotations to focus on skill development. Coach, take into consideration the pace of basketball games. It is detrimental to immolate an efficient sequence of drills in practices to give players a true game experience.

A discussion of the specific drills to be covered during this time is key to providing the athletes an opportunity to begin visualizing themselves executing the drills effectively. Begin with a series of dynamic warm-up drills that consist of calisthenics, plyometrics, and flexibility drills. These drills should identify the necessary concepts like footwork, body control, body positioning, and injury prevention. Progress to transition drills that emphasize speed change, agility, quickness, and explosiveness with efficiency. Provide athletes with time to recover, hydrate, and communicate any correction needed or answer questions before beginning skill-specific drills.

Some of the specific drills used will be based on the time of the season, the needs of the team, and the overall successful execution of the skill as a team. For example, ball handling, shooting, footwork, defense, offensive angles, and cuts are specific game breakdown drills. The duration of the drills depends on several factors: Full court or half-court typically will be approximately 8-10 minutes. If there are stations for the specific skill, it should be a 5-minute rotation. Timing for drills should consider the proper execution and confidence of each player. It is important that coaches not be afraid to sacrifice a little extra time on skill development to ensure the transfer of learning for proper game execution.

After the skills breakdown session, the application of skills in game pace drills is formatted to demonstrate and provide a visual of what and how those skills should be used. Some drills used are full court 5 player weave to 3 on 2, half court 4 on 4, and the 11-Man Drill.

Team practices will vary from week to week. Pre-season practice is built on strength and conditioning, preparing the body and mind for the season, proper nutrition, injury prevention, and recovery. This is when verbal instruction is at its heaviest to ensure expectations are known and embedded in each athlete.

The strength and conditioning program will encompass endurance running, like the 1.5-mile run, full-court, and half-court sprint work.

I also love to include pyramid sprints to build endurance and stamina, such as the 8-6-4-2 Drill. In this drill, athletes will run the width of the court sideline to sideline, beginning with 8 across and back in 45 seconds, six across and back in 35 seconds. Four across and back in 24 seconds, and 2 across and back in 12 seconds. Additionally, weight room workouts with free weights and machines to ensure good muscle development and strength.

A SAMPLE WEEK MAY LOOK LIKE THIS:

MONDAY: Endurance 1.5-mile timed, 200-meter and 100-meter sprints followed by walking lunges, standing squats, push-ups, and abdominal/core work.

TUESDAY: Footwork and plyometrics. Weight room upper body workout.

WEDNESDAY: 1.5-mile run. Lower body weight room workout.

THURSDAY: Ball handling, footwork, and passing drills, including sprint work and bodyweight conditioning at the end of practice.

The in-season strength and conditioning program will adjust to ensure rest and recovery and game-ready preparations. Weight training will continue; however, it will be adjusted to 3 days a week with more stretching and flexibility exercises and bodyweight exercises like pull-ups, push-ups, dips, and core work. Machine weight training instead of free weights ensures proper technique and alignment for good muscle development. Nutrition will be a year around awareness because it is important to efficient and productive game execution and preparation. The off-season program is most important. During the off-season, a complete review of the season will take place, and every area of the program should be addressed, and practice plans should reflect weaknesses of individual athletes, the team, and the overall program.

Variations, drills, efficient use of practice time, and on the court and off the court instruction are important to a successful team practice. Communication amongst athletes and their teammates and coaches is vital. Classroom instruction, breaking down film and play-by-play discussion is a must, especially during in-season. Pre–season videotaping is a good idea to help with skill development and execution. For example, have the athlete see himself or herself performing a skill and provide corrective feedback. Instruction needs to be specific to what the team is doing or not doing, not the competition. Practice time must be effective and efficient; always have an agenda with drills and times listed.

A SAMPLE PRACTICE PLAN IS FOUND BELOW:

6:30: 200 jumps with jump rope

- 15 form shots in the paint (block, block, middle)
- 10 Free-throws

6:45: AGILITY/ WARMUP

- High knees
- Butt kicks
- Skips (small)
- Skips (big)
- Two feet stutter steps
- Karaoke
- Defensive slides slow to half them pick up

speed

- Sprint and backpedal
- Sprint/backpedal/drop step
- Lean and rock

6:55: STATIONS [5-MINUTE STATIONS]

- Boxing out/Rebounding
- Getting Open
- 3-on-3 help & recover
- Defensive closeout

7:15: TEAM DRILLS

- 3-Player Weave/5-Player Weave (3-on-2)
- Olympic shooting drill
- 4-on-4

7:30: TEAM DRILLS [CONTINUED]

- Press Break
- 4 across
- 2-2-1

7:45: 7 SHOT SERIES

7:55: CONDITIONING

- 8–6–4–2
- 35–sec Line Drill

8:00: TEAM FREE THROWS

COACHING BEHAVIORS

Often the best teachers are coaches. The methods and strategies used in a classroom are often used on the court and on the field. The ability to capture the attention of the athletes daily is vital to the success of a program. Voice is typically the choice; however, it tends to require adjustments depending on the athlete one is speaking to, the location, time, or situation. Coach, each player has a different temperament and different tolerance levels. One player might be motivated by the voice method, while another may shut down.

Once using the whistle is a constant connection and expectation for most athletes. With the whistle, a coach can inform athletes how the whistle will be used at the beginning of the season. For example, one long blow is, "stop what you are doing, stand at attention." Three quick blows could be, "time to go and collect all equipment." A short blow could be, "I see you, please stop." Providing athletes with a set daily routine will enhance focus because the expectation is known. The ability to make practices engaging and exciting to everyone involved is a strategy that must be mastered in order to hold attention. Athletes love the hype and attention of sports, the pep rallies, the fans cheering in the stands, and winning. Ensuring that all athletes feel valuable to the team/program is important. This can be achieved by making sure each player has a voice and the liberty to just have fun.

All athletes are not wired the same way. As a transformational coach, one should be able to identify the fast learners and the slow learners and have plans in place to accommodate those needs effectively without sacrificing anyone's dignity. Coaches consistently adjust plays to prevent or engage in games; this same mentality needs to be exhibited when instructing individual athletes. For example, grouping students who learn at a slower pace is not a good idea. Who will push them to do more and provide confidence? Peer-to-peer training and instruction can have an amazing impact on an athlete's performance if placed in the right setting or group. I like to pair upperclassmen with lowerclassmen. This improves communication and comradery across the program. Coaches will need to communicate and plan practices with these accommodations in mind.

Sometimes we can focus too much on performance expectations and beating the clock. We must ensure that all athletes understand and demonstrate the correct skills and techniques. As a coach, it is easy to get caught up in practices. Therefore, when it comes to learning and performance, a coach's practice structure is vital to those expectations. Creating practice plans that are inclusive of modifications and adjustments for specific athletes demonstrates true leadership.

It is imperative that head coaches meet regularly with their staff to ensure team performance goals are being met and individual athletes' abilities are being groomed and enhanced. These meetings should address the necessary adjustments needed to be made and the expectations required from all staff to prevent poor performance or behavior issues. Consequently, providing a place where athletes are given the opportunity to develop into positive young men and women with a positive self-image and a desire to be leaders for future generations.

GROWTH AND WELL-BEING OF ATHLETES

Being a head coach requires building and fostering relationships with people of various socioeconomic backgrounds, beliefs, and talents. To build a successful program, a head coach must first identify the types of athletes acquired. A coach must consider all athletes' psychological, physiological, emotional, spiritual, and academic development. Once the identification is made, the next step is to receive buy-in and trust of the program's vision. Building and fostering relationships with those athletes creates the bond that provides for assurance of a strong consideration for their growth and well-being.

Providing the proper training, conditioning, and nutrition in the pre-season is preferred to ensure the care and prevention of athletic injuries. In sports, we do not just play, we compete, which requires a higher level of physical strength and endurance. Students' financial situations vary. Some may not have access to fancy organic stores to help them make the healthiest choices possible.

Athletes come from various programs, and it is important as a head coach to express what methods will be required or not tolerated to ensure care and prevention of injuries. There should be a list of requirements for maintaining proper health and injury prevention in the athletes' handbook. The athletic trainer is the leader for all care and preventive measures, as he or she will be managing that prevention. However, it is the responsibility of the head coach to ensure those measurements are implemented, properly demonstrated, and administered to all athletes by all staff. Additionally, providing a safe and secure environment for athletes to train and staff that is certified in CPR/First Aid/AED, concussion protocols, strength and conditioning are key to preventing injuries. The Athletic Director must provide coaches the opportunity to acquire these certifications and ensure they can demonstrate and instruct athletes accordingly.

Coaches must be an example for their athletes, constantly demonstrating and modeling the appropriate behavior regarding sound chemical health. Every athlete will face those words of, "we need you faster, quicker, and stronger." Great coaches initiate that mindset with sound nutritional recommendations and specific performance training without the use of chemical substances. It is important that coaches address the issues of substance abuse, alcohol, drugs, and supplementation with their players and the dangers that may occur because of their use.

Expectations for players during the season, in the classroom, school, community, and off-season should be verbally discussed with parents and athletes at the beginning of the season. Additionally, the athletic handbook should be given to every athlete to take home and revisit those expectations with parents, and a signature form returned to the head coach. The head coach and his/her staff must emphasize what it means to represent one's school and community when participating in athletics. Players become leaders when they wear their uniforms. Uniforms allow players to stand out and become more than just the name on their back. No matter where they are, what time of the season, once an athlete, always an athlete, and that role comes at the cost of major expectations.

Strategies to change inappropriate attitudes and behaviors begin with everyone from the athletes to the staff understanding their roles and responsibilities. When people know their roles and expectations, they tend to behave differently. However, another strategy is to build positive relationships and get to know individual players. Pat Summit states, "The job was not about being a martinet. It was about preparing people to make good independent decisions. Getting them in the right spots at the right time was as much a matter of understanding them, and *talking* to them, as it was of directing their traffic" (Jenkins, 2013, pg. 144).

Often inappropriate attitudes and behaviors come from insecurities and prior uncomfortable situations. It is vital as a coach not to be afraid to let go and trust that athletes so often want to do the right thing. A good way is to limit the number of rules and have clear expectations and consequences for those expectations when not adhered to. Having athletes make the rules and consequences creates a more unified front where everyone can feel they have a voice. Surprisingly, each team I have coached selects the topic of tardiness to set the guidelines for. The consequence is running, which all of them hate to do.

Academics and athletics go hand in hand. The 'no pass, no play rule' is just having guidelines in place to ensure athletes are achieving the best grades is an empowering statement that says, "We care about student-athletes, and academic all-American athletes are what we strive to create." Some procedures to ensure athletes are students first are:

1. Having a weekly study hall in a computer lab or library to provide the academic environment for intellectual focus.

2. Having a specific grade that everyone must be at or above on progress reports or report cards regularly.

3. Communicating the importance of education and having a career after sports.

4. Providing an opportunity for athletes to volunteer at elementary schools to read and help younger students with their academics.

5. Rewarding athletes for their academic achievements at team meetings or before practice.

COACHING STAFF

A head coach must surround himself/herself with a staff that believes in serving others, possesses a love for his or her athletes, has a burning passion for coaching, and must be humble and transparent. Secondly, a head coach must have qualified coaches and have a strong sense of what it takes to be a successful coach, one that can inspire, train, and transform athletes.

To raise expertise within a coaching staff, head coaches must model the behaviors they wish to see. Coaches need to know and understand their responsibilities and expectations. This can be done with staff meetings, huddles, effective communication, and reviewing job descriptions. Providing the coaching staff with opportunities to attend professional development seminars, clinics, coaching certification, and degree programs like Concordia can also raise their level of expertise.

Meetings should be scheduled weekly to retain information, keep the vision clear, and make necessary adjustments to program happenings and player development.

Communication is key to the success of any business or organization. All staff must be "on the same page" daily to ensure proper guidance of the team—positive coaching vs. demanding behaviors. A line must be drawn when it comes to the proper deliverance of instructions, corrections, motivations, and constructive criticism. Joe Ehrmann's philosophy about being a transactional coach (demanding behaviors) or transformational coach (positive coaching) delivers a great message. Transactional coaching is stated to be characteristic of more self-centered coaches. They demand things from their players with no exceptions. They use their platform to generate a position of power for themselves, not for their athletes. Transactional coaches possess the "what can the player do for me" mentality. Their coaching techniques are about what it takes to win the game versus creating the kind of athlete with pride, character, and respect that would consistently develop into a winning tradition.

Ehrmann states that transactional coaches "operated on a quid pro quo basis to incentivize us to perform better, they looked for what they could get out of coaching and not what they could give; they ignored athletes' developmental needs and often manipulated and distorted the values of winning and losing" (Ehrmann, 2011, Pg. 7).

On the contrary, the transformational coach connects with their athletes and builds relationships that foster good character, values, and discipline. Transformational coaches care about their athletes' well-being; therefore, they are attuned to what is required to empower each athlete. Transformational coaches use their platform to demonstrate the appropriate actions, behaviors, and expectations of a successful program and athlete. A transformational coach is dedicated to self-understanding and empathy, viewing sports as a virtuous and virtue-giving discipline (Ehrmann, 2011, Pg. 6). As a transformational coach, there seems to be an easier road to success because the view is more about whom you are coaching, not what you are coaching.

As coaches, it is our duty to coach the game and instill greater values in our players. We are the carpenters chosen to build men and women of character that this world can respect. Therefore, when we see a football player, basketball player, volleyball player, soccer player, or baseball player, we see more than just an athlete.

Transformational coaching is a good tool of positive reinforcement for learning new skills and rewarding good player behavior because the focus is on the player, not just the performance. Additionally, with individual goal setting, motivational quotes, and tangible rewards, the quest for learning will generate better behaviors.

I like to incorporate videos to help motivate and inspire my players. I have discovered that they respond well to movies that feature teams overcoming challenges. Likewise, having teams participate in team-building activities and individually and collaboratively helping others can generate positive attitudes and alleviate unwanted behaviors. It is imperative that the head coach and his/her staff consistently demonstrate and communicate the importance of commitment, a sound work ethic, and the importance of having integrity. By combining all the above efforts, learning and behavior management will occur.

The assistant coach's primary responsibility is to identify the opposing team's strengths, weaknesses, and habits. It is important for the head coach to have qualified and capable assistants to break down film and data with the use of various software programs, like *Hudl* and *Athlete Monitoring.* Weekly game-planning meetings will help keep your staff sharp and identify strategies for upcoming games. Additionally, in these meetings, data from previous games can be assessed, post-game observations analyzed, player adjustments made if necessary, and other observations the staff may have noticed. Outside of video, of course, is the actual attendance of an opponent's games in the pre–season and during the season. On several occasions, I have taken my team to the local university to expose them to what possibilities lay before them. The impact echoed in their increased passion for the game and their improved performance in the classroom.

Teams grow, change, and adjust often; therefore, it is important to witness the change and adjustments and discuss those changes and how they will impact the team's performance.

Motivating individuals and teams is a personal endeavor that every head coach must consistently and collaboratively do with their coaching staff. Motivation tends to be easier when one has a relationship with an individual. Being consistent, firm, and fair with rules, policies, and procedures is a key component. Likewise, allow players to have a voice and create a family bond atmosphere, a safe space where disagreements and issues can arise, but everyone works together to solve them.

For example, regularly giving compliments, like "great job" or a pat on the back, to just say, "I see your efforts, keep it up." Pat Summit created a system where the player had to say "two points" out loud whenever she complimented them, whereas if she gave them criticism, they had to say "rebound," meaning shake it off, take the lesson, and then move on (Jenkins, 2013. Pg. 215). Motivation needs to be a collective engagement by all involved in one's program, it is by this effort that performance is enhanced, and team victories tend to occur.

CHARACTER DEVELOPMENT

An athlete with good character is coachable, has a great work ethic, works well with others, looks to always improve, perseveres, and is honest and loyal. An athlete with good character is not afraid to make sacrifices to better oneself or the team. Good character in an athlete permeates to others. Others see that athlete as more than just an athlete, but a person of integrity and a leader for future athletes, a mentor, a true friend.

A head coach must have in place as part of his/ her program the importance of having good character and the specific character traits that are important, and how to demonstrate and encourage their use. There are various programs that coaches and their staff can use, such as the Student–Athlete Program, Character and Leadership Development. With this program, athletes receive an online lesson via an interactive app on their devices seven days a week. The athletes' responses go directly to their coaches. Coaches will meet with athletes daily or weekly to discuss their daily lessons.

The program also provides team-building leadership exercises to strengthen team unity, drive, and cohesion. Consequently, Coaches must be the example of the character traits they wish to see. By modeling what they wish to see, athletes can have a mentor to ensure they are consistently the person their coaches hope for them to be.

When correcting or confronting a negative behavior, it is imperative that the response is to the behavior and not the athlete. Addressing the behavior itself is vital to its correction versus boldly and loudly addressing the athlete and causing them to feel humiliated. I let my players know that their choices will affect more than just their playing time. Timing of the correcting of the behavior is important, and knowledge of the athlete is important as well. Coaches must be considerate of these aspects. A coach's response to behaviors must be consistent with their prior communicated expectations, rules, policies, and procedures.

There will be times when a coach may need to remove a player from practice, dismiss a player from a game, or remove a player from the team. This should only occur if the athlete deliberately went against an established written rule or expectation. The athlete should be provided an opportunity to correct the behavior or rectify the situation. If the behavior is a true violation of the league's rules or policies outlined in the athletic handbook or considered unethical, the process of removal should be followed as stated in the handbook. It is important for the protection of the program that the head coach addresses these types of situations immediately and document all verbal communication and actions taken.

Removing a player from practice typically

sends a message that their behavior was inappropriate, not going to be tolerated, or was hurting the team. In this instance, the behavior will take care of itself. However, the behavior must be addressed immediately, and a means of correction must be provided or adhered to. Communication with the team at the close of the practice of the incident must be initiated to prohibit further discussion that may generate a negative response between players and or coaches. A call or meeting with parents should be done immediately. This protects the head coach's integrity and prevents any miscommunication of the situation. Whether on the phone or in person, be sure to stick to the specifics of the situation. Address the behavior, not the athlete. Note any rules or expectations that were not adhered to and the consequences thereof. Provide and or discuss a plan of action on how the player can improve his or her behavior. Send an email to the athlete's parent informing them about the meeting and what was discussed, and the plan of action. Finally, place a copy in the athlete's file.

Removing a player from a team is always

the last resort. Great head coaches know the importance of creating change in athletes and understand that being an athlete is a choice, and it requires an immense amount of time, dedication, and sacrifice. Furthermore, they can create programs inclusive of individuals from various socioeconomic areas, ethnicities, cultures, talents, and personalities. If a player is to be removed from a team, it must be justifiable, and there must be clear evidence of inappropriate misbehaviors that are unethical or have willfully defied team or program rules or policies. Every effort should be made to keep the player on the team and provide any necessary resources to ensure the future success of that player. Joe Ehrmann states, "He believes that coaching should build character, not focus on the extrinsic motivators like the ultimate prizes of being an athlete; money, sex, fame or more professionally termed, validation, status, and identity. Furthermore, it should transform the athlete's lives to ensure future success as young men and women" (Ehrmann, 2011, Pg. 57).

As a head coach, one should never compromise the integrity of the team, their values, and their code of ethics. Behaviors that undermine established rules, policies, procedures, and program expectations should not be compromised. Athletes must adhere to a coach's program expectations, and if they find that they are unable to do so, it is in the best interest of that program that they be excused. One athlete can change the dynamics of a program if allowed.

True athletes view rules as challenges. They do not break them, they rise above them. It is important that a head coach secures a solid buy-in from every team member. Establishing and building relationships is a key component because those who know your vision and understand your expectations will not request a compromise at any time. A transformational coach considers every aspect of an athlete, their social, physical, mental, and emotional state of mind, not just their talent or exceptional athletic ability.

The qualities of a great team and the strategies to mold them into a single unit come from the vision and expectations of the head coach. First, the vision must be clear, understood, and accepted, as should the expectations. All members involved feel that they can fulfill the vision and play an integral part in its mission. Secondly, head coaches must show that they can coordinate these differences to create their vision. Thirdly, the identification of the role and responsibilities of everyone must be clearly defined and obtainable, and a tailored plan generated for achievement. Being a great team is having a true sense of pride in the organization one represents, wanting to do well not just for yourself but also for the program, total loyalty, respecting other differences and celebrating the smallest of improvements, treating every member like family and enjoying every moment of the journey together.

FUNDRAISING AND BOOSTERS

There is a constant battle to secure funding for school-based programs. Time and time again, I have seen fundraisers and booster supporters provide economic leverage for athletics. Head coaches must be familiar with the policies and procedures for the various fundraising opportunities and the school/district policies and procedures on the collection of monies.

Fundraising brings a community effort to athletic programs and generates a sense of pride and belonging for athletes. Some popular programs, like Deanon Gourmet Popcorn, Ultimate Dining Card, Charity Auctions, and Host a tournament, generate quick collections and do not require additional work for coaches and staff.

The booster club is an organization formed by parents to support an associate club, sports team, or organization. Their support is based on fundraising or coordinating various events for that program. A booster club provides funding for the programs that are not receiving enough funds to supply equipment, uniforms, coaching staff, awards, and banquets. Additionally, booster clubs can provide a means of management for funds collected, ensuring that the program has everything it needs to run successfully. Booster Clubs are an opportunity for parents to become involved in athletic programs and get a clear understanding of the needs of the athletic programs and ensure that those programs are successful and provide a quality program to their athletes.

BUILDING RELATIONSHIPS

Team involvement in the community and service-learning is instrumental to the development of athletes during and after their sports careers. Community involvement provides a sense of well-being and teaches athletes the importance of helping others. Habitat for Humanity is a great organization where teams can connect with those organizers to build homes for families. Spending a day at a children's cancer center provides athletes with a caring heart and an understanding of what resiliency can truly mean. The head coach can select a game night to invite special needs students to stand with the players or have the athletes collect toys to give to families in shelters for Christmas. Building relationships with community outreach is a learning experience that creates freedom and a desire to forever serve others.

Parents have a major effect on athletic programs. It is the most important entity that a head coach must deal with regularly. To build relationships with parents, a coach must communicate often and consistently. A coach must keep parents informed of the role and expectations of their child. It is imperative that coaches outline their vision and expectations for the program and each individual athlete to the parents. This may include, but is not limited to, game-day rules, practices, player rotations, and outside-of-game expectations.

Additionally, coaches should be specific about their parents' expectations and what they will not accept or tolerate from them. For example, time and place to discuss their son/daughter playing time or position during a game. Parents should be reminded of their role as supporters of their children and the athletic program and the importance of ensuring positive reports and uplifting and assisting the program whenever necessary.

Communication with parents should encompass more positives than negatives. Assistant coaches can be beneficial in communicating with parents and providing feedback about their son/daughter. With the use of technology, such as email, Remind, and other apps, coaches can conveniently communicate regularly to parents without handouts or letters. Communication is the key to successful relationships. For coaches, it is the glue that holds programs together and keeps them functioning smoothly, and the lack thereof can tear them apart.

Head coaches must consider all the aforementioned aspects to have a successful program. It is important to begin with a vision that includes staff, players, the district, and the community. The focus should be on transforming lives through sports, not wins and losses. Wins will come when you build strong relationships and buy into the vision. Consequently, the approach taken must be of confidence and humility because to transform programs and lives, one must be willing to sacrifice a bit of oneself. Great Coaches inspire, motivate, and uplift others and create an environment that fosters positive relationships and builds future leaders for today's society. A program of that caliber will have a legacy.

CHAPTER VII
PSYCHOLOGY OF COACHING

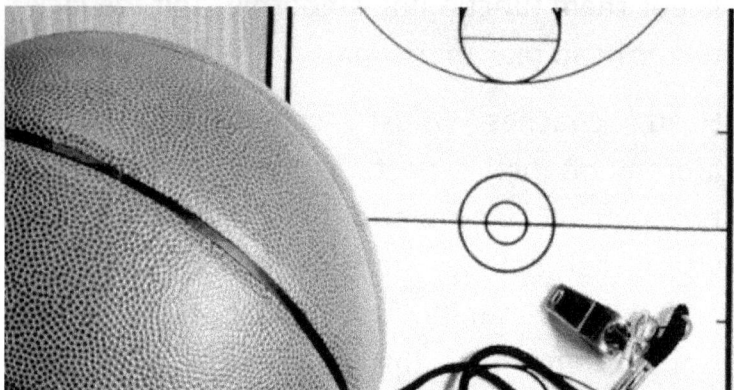

The principles of psychology can be applied in every facet of a coaching environment. To build positive relationships with their staff and players, head coaches must understand the importance and effectiveness of implementing those principles. Considering the techniques can assist with the social aspects and the emotional. Consequently, providing a means of behavior management can undoubtedly be an issue with athletes.

There are a variety of principles for coaches to consider. The techniques can be used collaboratively or individually, based on the needs of the program. For example, setting goals can create a clearer vision of where we are and where we would like to be. According to Locke and Latham, there is an inseparable link between goal setting and workplace performance. Their theory on goal–setting justifies the need for it in sports.

The basic premise of this research is that an individual's conscious ideas regulate his actions. Studies are cited demonstrating that: 1) hard goals produce a higher level of performance (output) than easy goals, 2) specific hard goals produce a higher level of output than a goal of "do your best," and 3) behavioral intentions regulate choice behavior. The theory also views goals and intentions as mediators of the effects of incentives on task performance (Locke, 1968).

Like goal setting, having good communications skills is crucial to building positive relationships. According to situation or circumstance, a head coach must take pride in delivering messages to staff and players limitedly and appropriately. As noted – Mental Training Program, players need to know how to positively communicate or articulate their words without demeaning, being negative, or tearing someone down. Also, they need to know how to express themselves appropriately in any given situation. Head coaches and their staff fall under this umbrella, as well. Communication is a joint venture for everyone in the program, and it must be a priority for the head coach to have expectations set forth and be an example of what he or she wants to hear.

According to Alan Tsz Lun, cohesion is multi-dimensional, including task cohesion, which is the level of unity in task performance (e.g., teamwork and task completion within sports such as working together to win a championship). Secondly, there is social cohesion which is the level of unity in social aspects (e.g., social support and friendships outside of sports). As a head coach, these two dimensions will play vital roles in a team's performance. Providing opportunities for players to collaborate on practice agendas, game strategies, and ensuring that everyone has a voice and feels part of the program, is instrumental in building team cohesion.

There are strategies or techniques that can be used to determine the cohesiveness of a team, such as a questionnaire, a survey, or individual meetings with players. In sports, the one affects the whole.

Once the level of team cohesiveness has been determined, strategies should be implemented immediately to improve team cohesion. Some specific areas to target are team environment, team structure, team processes, and team climate. Team cohesion must be identified early to negate any relationship or behavior issues. A good time for implementation is pre-season. Continue to monitor it weekly to ensure everyone carries out those expectations for the entire season.

Stress management, relaxation techniques or concentration, and control strategies must be implemented, encouraged, or regularly displayed. Sports tend to elude behaviors often misinterpreted as out of control versus intense, passionate, or excited. As a head coach, those behaviors must be addressed and identified as to what is appropriate and what is not. Likewise, the importance of self-awareness and self-confidence must be addressed as well. Understanding how to cope with wins and losses, having a bad game, being "that great player," and the pressures that come with being an athlete must be discussed, acknowledged, and consistently addressed daily. Providing opportunities for players to get away, take a break from practices by going on field trips, helping others, or just spending time talking about things other than sports can help manage personal stress levels. Head coaches may also encourage advice seeking through athletic counselors, informational gatherings, planning, problem-solving, and proactive behaviors to maintain a balanced mental and emotional state

Coaching the game is different from coaching/teaching players. Therefore, when it comes to working with others, it requires a sense of psychological knowledge and a willingness to evaluate other beliefs, behaviors, and ways of communicating. Creating an environment that is conducive to learning and provides consistent opportunities for growth and development is expected of a transformational leader. Treating players like human beings and not just athletes can bring greatness to any program.

CHAPTER VIII
ATS FOR COACHING BASKETBALL

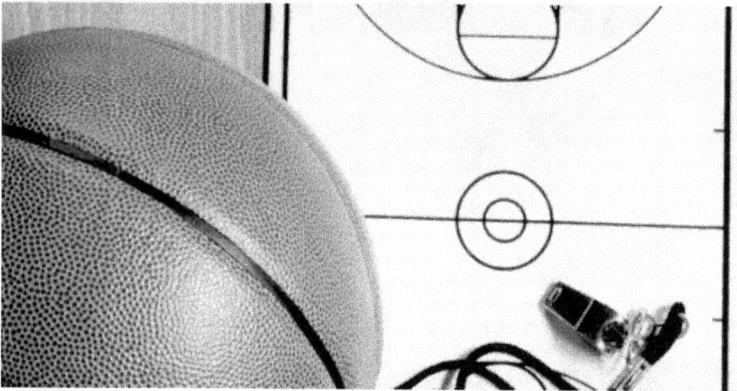

As a high school, collegiate, and semi-professional student-athlete, experiencing many different coaching styles is not uncommon. As an assistant coach, learning various skillsets based on the head coach's philosophy helps create a vision and philosophy of one's own. Through these experiences, one can learn what works and does not work with offensive and defensive schemes, in addition to program development and player development. As a head coach, building a program where everyone is involved, from the coaching staff to the players, is the focus.

Ensuring that everyone involved has a clear understanding of the coaching vision and philosophy and using their talents to create a program that everyone is proud to be a part of within that vision. A program where there is collaboration and decision making, where no one is afraid to express an idea or a thought. Creating an environment that has expectations and standards, and all talents/skills are known, encouraged, and respected.

As a coach, one will witness programs where parents dictate who plays and when to get rid of the coach, based on what they think is not happening, according to what they feel or think they know better. I have resolved this issue in my program by hosting a parent's practice. This allows the parents to become familiar with the plays and policies of the game.

I have been on teams where a coach only plays their top seven players. Why recruit them if they are not going to play at least half the time every year of their career? Having to witness coaches not teaching their athletes the fundamentals of the game but expecting to win with that one good player is disheartening. The experience of being athletic enough to make the roster but lacking the skills to play a specific position and get in the game is a bit hard to swallow. I imagine: Why didn't those previous coaches teach us all the skills to play every position?

So often, teams set goals, individually and collectively. Personally, goals are important for individual achievement because it helps with accountability and focus. However, team goals should be few and simple. For example: Be the best version of yourself you can be. Be kind to others. Be willing to make sacrifices. Stay committed and in the moment.

Gregg Popovich's video on the Spurs' Philosophy System Basics speaks to what is important within a team. He states, "It is more about organization, discipline, building the blocks, and relationships with your players… all these things have more to do with winning and losing than being able to draw a certain play." He believes that "They am, what they am, and often we cannot change that, therefore that player may have to go. The fiber of your team is the beginning of everything that you do" (Popovich, 2016).

Character is who you are, no matter where you are. Student–athletes are to be men and women of great character that are leaders, not just athletes. I am not the type of coach to sacrifice character for skill level. All student–athletes will be held to the same standards of honesty, great character, a strong sense of drive and initiative, respect for the game, themselves, and others. There will be no big I's and little you's; everyone will be held accountable in the same manner, from the bench player to the star player.

OFFENSIVE PRINCIPLES/SYSTEM

Offensive principles have a way of defining your program. It is often the first thing noticed by potential athletes. There is much admiration for a coach who can create an offense with multiple strategies that allow athletes to fit into the system and produce results. The preferred offensive principles are up–tempo, have lots of ball movement, and are focused on a high percentage shot selection. High percentage scoring is important because it opens other opportunities for rebounds, put–backs, and free throws. A motion offense is preferred because of more scoring opportunities for all players. A quick hitter offense removes stagnation. Movement away from that ball is key to ensure spacing and play development.

With this type of offense, we are looking to pass more, set screens, and move the ball without dribbling. However, the dribble drive and kick is very effective within this type of offense. The transition from defense tends to flow better into the offense without a formal setup. This type of offensive system will require a focus on individual skill development because it allows players to be creative within a semi-structured setting. Additionally, it helps diversify the post player by moving from the block to transitioning to more short corner baseline jumpers to three-pointers and high post moves off the dribble.

Some of the sets that work well with this type of offensive system are the 4-low, double-stack guard/post, 4-out, or the high-low when playing against a zone defense. With every offense, there are weaknesses. If players are afraid or hesitant about shooting or moving without the ball, it will defeat the offense. Secondly, if the guards are uncomfortable driving to the basket, communicating these things verbally may cause a breakdown in the offensive set. Furthermore, it requires knowing your teammates and how they play and trusting the system.

We want to be aggressive when going to the basket, and we are looking for a fast break opportunity, working the angles and coming off the screens tight and low, ready to score. Being familiar with a variety of screens—down, up, back door, double, ball, off-the-ball—and being able to execute those properly is key. Therefore, when we practice, it is a breakdown of its parts because the development of fundamentals to ensure precise execution is crucial. Skill development is the focus of my practices. The select type of drills emphasized are teaching student-athletes about setting screens, jump-stops, getting open, movement without the ball, dribbling, passing, and offensive rebounding. This system tends to be most effective; however, it is not set in stone. Creating different sets out of this offensive system based on the type of talent given for that season or what opponent we may be facing at that moment generates its effectiveness or not.

DEFENSIVE PRINCIPLES/SYSTEM

The saying that "offense fills the seats, but defense wins games" is true. Pat Summit built one of the best programs in Tennessee.

She states that "Offense sells tickets, defense wins games, rebounding wins championships." Her principles for defense are relevant and just. For her team, "the core principles of defense and rebounding are continually stressed in pre-practice talks, worked on in drills, reinforced with coaching, and reprimanded with team running when someone forgets to do them. They are also discussed and monitored before, during, and after games" (Hansen, 2016).

As a collegiate student-athlete, defense is my preference. Being blessed with great speed and a 31" vertical, rebounding and steals came easy. With every game, the mission was to dominate on the boards and provide as many fast-break opportunities for our team as possible. Fortunately, the coaches saw the talent and used it. As a coach today, defense is the focus. Defense wins games, but it also fuels the teams' energy and passion for the game. Not every player likes to play defense. Most players do not because it takes work and comes from within. Defensive skills can be taught, but the execution must be learned, accepted, and regularly practiced to the point that it is automatically played accordingly.

The basketball defensive principles and system would be considered a combination defense. Altering or changing defenses by possessions keeps the offense guessing. With defensive alignments, a half-man, half-zone defense versus a straight-up man-to-man defense is preferred. Defense is more effective when everyone contributes to getting defensive stops. For example, closing out is a struggle for some players. They tend to want to jump into the offensive player, coming off the ground and allowing dribble penetration. Having that help defense available is important to stopping that movement and playing a 3–2 zone set with trapping on the perimeters. Again, it requires teamwork and knowledge of those concepts of help and recovery, fronting the post, denying, and others.

Full court is not a driving force for my defense. It opens the door for mishaps and free-scoring opportunities. Preferably a quarter-court defense leads into a defensive set and allows for a more secure help and recovery. With this defensive system, we can focus more on creating mistakes for the offense than forcing steals to happen haphazardly. Defensively we should be taking away opportunities and forcing immediate change in another's offense, which leads to turnovers, deflection, and defensive stops.

When the ball is under the basket or on the sidelines, defensive play is where the knowledge of defensive principles is key. When teaching the proper skills and fundamentals of defense, those situations truly highlight a student-athletes lack of defensive skill set. One-on-one defense is my favorite skill to teach because the footwork, intensity, body positioning, and spacing is consistently challenged when playing defense. Consequently, in these situations, one on one defensive skill development is put into play. In our practices, we focus a lot on the basic concepts of defensive skills. For example, hand positioning when defending, denying the ball, defensive stance, blocking out and rebounding, playing the ball, help and recovery, and trapping.

When teaching defense, it is a day of practice solely devoted to its mastery. Creating an environment full of energy with drills that are competitive and push the student–athletes to their fullest potential is key. We do station work to break down the skills to ensure every student–athlete executes it effectively and efficiently as one unit when they come together on the court. We invest a lot of seconds on the foundational skills with defensive stations, offensive stations, and rebounding stations to create muscle memory within the player. Make sure to keep these drills challenging and energetic to keep the players from becoming stagnant. These drills are also a great opportunity to teach players how to move without the ball. We focus on each part of the game to help the players understand it.

In conclusion, over time, the abilities and talents

of athletes change, and as coaches, we should adjust. Being reluctant to system changes and adjustments is common with coaches; however, with professional development and experience, one soon realizes that things and people change and adjustments are okay. When the system is effective, and the student-athletes are having fun, the adjustments were well worth it.

CHAPTER IX
AT THE BUZZER

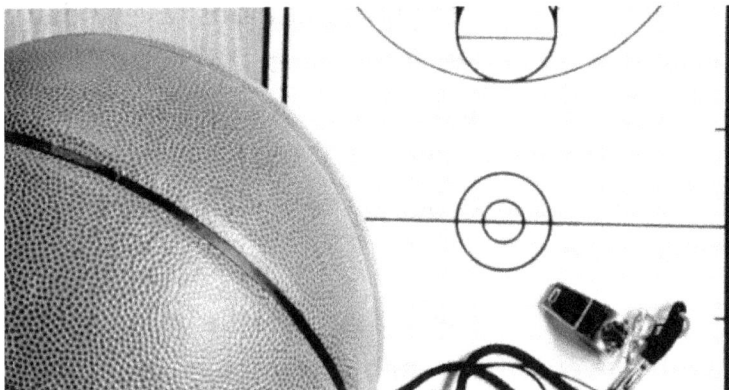

Some experiences sometimes need to be forgotten. Then there are those experiences that grow and mature you in many ways. Having the opportunity to consider sports and athletics with a Christian-based view, with a thoroughness that goes deeper than just coaching, and a reality that places my life in perspective is invaluable. Likewise, the opportunity to look within me and evaluate my past experiences in coaching and acknowledge who I truly am as a person and a coach has been enlightening. Thanks to Jeffrey Marx's book, *Season of Life*, I have discovered that

I am a transformational leader and a type-A personality when it comes to coaching and teaching athletes. I am driven and passionate about seeing others reach their highest potential. There are no limitations. Every day is a day to grow, learn, and do more than required to be the best at anything. The future of my student-athletes will continue to be my focus, with sports being the vehicle that drives their journey.

By becoming leaders that provide more than skill development and strategies for their programs, coaches can enhance their careers as well as their student-athletes. My greatest joy was getting the opportunity to see Joe Ehrmann in person after reading his story. It brought everything to light with my personal vision as a coach. I wanted everyone to know him and read his story, both coaches and student-athletes.

I realized that I am happiest when coaching and around athletes and other coaches. Being in this program has provided the vision for the next journey: Head Coach or Athletic Director. Furthermore, I discovered that there were some things I was completely unfamiliar with, like the true importance of scouting, booster clubs, and the importance of understanding the logistics of funding and financial obligations within athletics, from bids to facility management, risk management, and the processes to ensure successful athletic programs. Not to mention the importance of knowing sports law.

In conclusion, I grace this book with the blessing of being seen by an Athletic Director who is inspired by my vision, my passion for sports, and my love for student-athletes, that they will encourage their coaches to read this book.

COACH G STATS

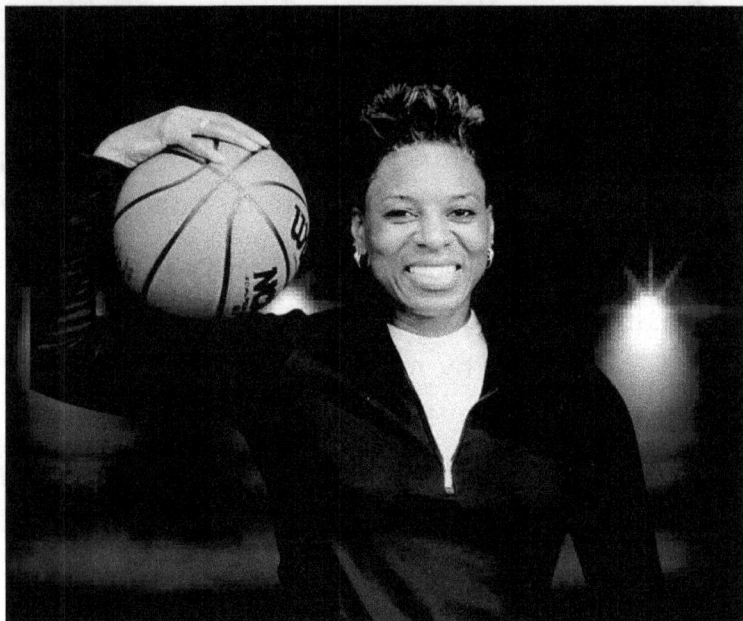

Thomasina 'Coach G' Gatson

29 YEARS OF EXPERIENCE

VP OF TAHPERD

HEALTH TEACHER OF THE YEAR

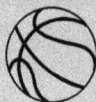

TWO-TIME DISTRICT FINALIST

SECONDARY TEACHER OF THE YEAR

Associates of Arts in Physical Education
Bachelor of Science in Kinesiology
Masters in Education of Administration
Masters in Business Administration
Masters in Coaching Administration
Sports Specific Trainer

Thomasina "Coach G" Gatson always knew the play for her life involved basketball and coaching players of the future. The squeak of sneakers against hardwood floors is the soundtrack to her life. Her sneakers have graced every court in her career, from middle school to collegiate to professional. Basketball has always been a haven for her, a defense of peace against chaos. Coach G has dribbled past distractions for the past twenty-nine years to reach her personal improvement and student-athlete development goals. Her passion for health and our youth has led her to open her sports performance academy, Gatson's Fitness & Sports Academy, to teach the game of basketball and help students secure funds for college.

References- Appendix B

ACE Blog. (2016). *Coach's Corner: Coach Wooden's Example.* Retrieved on January

    21, 2017.

Aldine Independent School District. School Messenger Presence. Retrieved January 11,

2018, from http://www.aldineisd.org

Ardoy, D.N., J. M. Fernandez-Rodriguez, D. Jimenez-Pavon, R. Castillo, J. R. Ruiz,

F. B. Ortega. (2014). A Physical Education trial improves adolescents' cognitive

performance and academic achievement: the EDUFIT study. *Scandinavian*

Journal of Medicine & Science in Sports, 24, 52-61.

Arons, Abigail. (2011). Childhood Obesity in Texas: The Cost, The Policies, and a

Framework for the Future. The Children's Hospital Association of Texas.

    32.

Atkinson, Russell (2015). Does physical activity improve academic performance?

Physical and Health Education Journal, 80 (4), 22–23.

Castelli, Darla M., Elizabeth Glowacki, Jeanne M. Barcelona, Hanna G. Calvert &

Jungyun Hwang. (2015). Active Education: Growing evidence on physical

activity and academic performance. *Active Living Research*. Research Brief. 1–5. Accessed from www.activelearningresearch.org.

Centers for Disease Control and Prevention, (2010). The association between school-based physical activity, including physical education, and academic performance. Atlanta, Ga: U.S. Department of Health and Human Services.

Chu, Tsz Lun. (2017). *From "Me" to "We": Promoting Team Cohesion among Youth*

Athletes.

Association for Applied Sports Psychology. Parent and Youth Sports. University of North Texas; AASP Youth Sport SIG.

Cotton, D.J. & Wolohan, J.T. – *Law for Recreation*

and Sport Managers, 6th Edition.

Kendall/ Hunt Publishing: Dubuque, Iowa p. 78–79.

Delgado, Richard. (2014). Coaches Athletic Handbook. Retrieved January 11, 2018,

from http://www.aldineisd.org University Interscholastic League. (2018). University of Texas at Austin. Retrieved January 11, 2018, from http://www.uiltexas.org

Ehrmann, J, Ehrmann, P. & Jordan G. (2011). *InSideOut Coaching: How Sports Can Transform Lives*. Simon & Schuster. New York, NY.

Fletcher, Molly. (2014). *5 Core Values Behind Pat Summits' Legendary Leadership.*

The Molly Fletcher Company. Retrieved from

https://mollyfletcher.com/5-core-values-behind-pat-summit-legendary-leadership.

Holmes, Venita, Dr. PH. (2010). Correlation and predictive analysis of obesity on student

Achievement using HISD Fitness Gram results, 2008–2009. Research and

Accountability Department. (3) 2. 2–9.

Jenkins, Sally. (2013). *Sum It Up Pat Summit.* Crown Publishing Group, Random House, Inc., New York.

Locke, Edwin. (1968). *Toward a theory of task motivation and incentives.*

Organizational Behavior and Human Performance. Elsevier Inc.

Lumpkin, A., Stoll, S. K., & Beller, J.M. (2012). *Practical ethics in sport management.* Jefferson, NC: McFarland.

Martens, R. (2004). *Successful Coaching*, 4th Ed., Champaign, IL: Human Kinetics.

Marx, J. (2003). *Season of life; A football star, a boy, a journey to manhood.* New York, NY: Simon & Schuster.

Meadors, L. Ph.D. (2017). *Practical Application for Long-Term Athletic Development.*

National Strength and Conditioning Association. P. 6.

Texas Education Agency. (2015). *Physical Education (PE) and Physical Activity (PA)*

Frequently asked Questions. Education Service Center Region 12.

Trost, S. and Van Der Mars, H. (2009). Why we should not cut P.E. *Educational Leadership*. (67) 2. 60.

Williamson, Marianne. Poem. A Return to Love: Reflections on the Principles of "A Course in Miracles."

www.ingramcontent.com/pod-product-compliance
Lightning Source LLC
Chambersburg PA
CBHW060645150426
42811CB00085B/2418/J